Everything You Need to Know About

Vision
Disorders

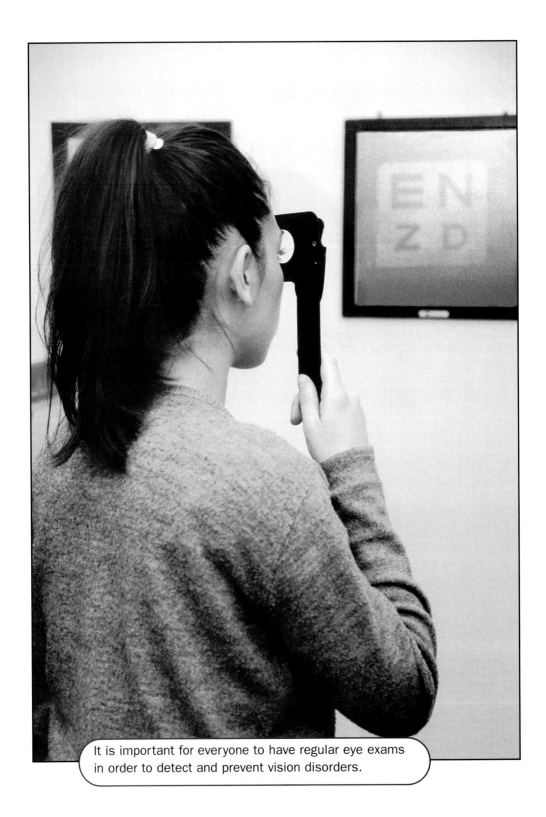

It is important for everyone to have regular eye exams in order to detect and prevent vision disorders.

Everything You Need to Know About

Vision Disorders

Debbie Stanley

The Rosen Publishing Group, Inc.
New York

Published in 2001 by The Rosen Publishing Group, Inc.
29 East 21st Street, New York, NY 10010

Library of Congress Cataloging-in-Publication Data

Stanley, Debbie.
Everything you need to know about vision disorders / by Debbie Stanley. —1st ed.
   p. cm. —(The need to know library)
Includes bibliographical references (p.) and index.
Summary: Discusses some of the disorders that may affect a person's vision, their symptoms and treatments, and the importance of visiting an eye doctor.
   ISBN 0-8239-3225-7 (library binding)
   1. Vision disorders—Juvenile literature. [1. Vision disorders.] I. Title. II. Series.
   RE52 .S73 20000
   617.7—dc21

                             00-008725

Manufactured in the United States of America

Contents

	Introduction	6
Chapter One	**Less-than-Perfect Vision**	9
Chapter Two	**Take Action: Don't Ignore**	
	These Problems	17
Chapter Three	**Emergency!**	
	Get Help Now	35
Chapter Four	**Protecting Your Sight**	42
	Glossary	55
	Where to Go for Help	58
	For Further Reading	61
	Index	62

Introduction

Many people think of sight as their most precious sense. Being without it in daily life is very limiting: You can't drive a car, you can't read street signs, you can't see sunsets or people's faces. Because sight is so valuable, the thought of losing it to an injury or disease can be very frightening. However, it is important to know that many of the causes of poor vision or even blindness can be prevented.

There are many, many diseases and conditions that can affect your vision. Some start in the eye itself, while others start in the brain. Some vision problems are painful, while others are not. They may have very obvious symptoms, or subtle symptoms, or no symptoms at all. Some vision disorders cause immediate, dramatic changes to your vision, while others start slowly and gradually become worse. Some vision disorders lead to complete blindness, while others are temporary and will go away with treatment or by themselves.

In this book you will find information on many vision disorders, including what symptoms to look for and how problems can be treated or avoided.

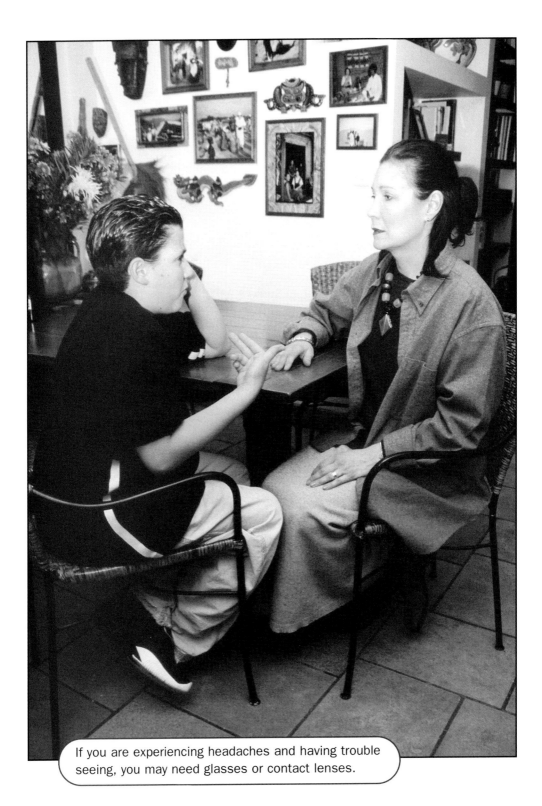

If you are experiencing headaches and having trouble seeing, you may need glasses or contact lenses.

Chapter One

Less-than-Perfect Vision

*A*s Carter sits in his chemistry class, his head pounds. His eyes burn. Carter tries to pay attention because chemistry is his favorite class. Normally, when Ms. Schell mixes different chemicals together to show their reaction, he is so intrigued he can barely sit still. It amazes him how some chemicals when mixed together not only explode but flash vibrant colors.

Lately though, Ms. Schell could be demonstrating how to make pure gold and Carter would not care. His head hurts so badly each day, he can only lay it down on his desk and close his eyes. His grades are getting lower with each passing week because he can never pay attention.

Carter knows he has to do something, and he knows what he has to do: He must tell his mother that he needs glasses. He can no longer see the blackboard and he sits in only the third row. His friends wave to him in the hallway, but until he stands a few feet away from them, he doesn't know who is waving to him.

The problem is that Carter doesn't want to wear glasses. He's afraid that he will look like a nerd or a freak. But now that his grades are suffering, he knows he has to risk it.

That night at dinner, while Carter is eating his mashed potatoes, he blurts out, "Mom, I can't see anything anymore. I'm doing really badly in chemistry because my head hurts all the time. But I don't want glasses. I'll look stupid."

"OK. I'll make an appointment for you. As to your looking stupid, Carter, I know you're scared you'll look weird, but you are worrying way too much. We'll get you glasses that look great or maybe some contacts."

"You're right, Mom. I am worrying too much. And nothing could look worse than the safety goggles we have to wear in chemistry."

Vision problems are common among teens. In fact, lots of people wear glasses or contact lenses to improve their vision. More than 120 million Americans wear glasses or contact lenses, and over 25 percent of adults are nearsighted. However, many teens, when they find out they need glasses, begin to worry. Like Carter, they fear that others will tease them because of their new appearance. If you need glasses and you are scared or upset, talk to someone—a parent, a teacher, or even just a close friend—and try to find a solution, but don't cheat yourself out of seeing the world just because of other people's opinions.

There are two basic problems that could cause you to need glasses: nearsightedness and farsightedness. Nearsightedness, also called myopia, makes it hard for a person to see things that are far away from them. Depending on how severe their nearsightedness, they might have trouble reading street signs, seeing the blackboard in school, or even seeing things on the floor at their feet, but they usually have no trouble seeing the print in a book held in their hands.

Farsightedness is less common among younger people. It can be caused either by hyperopia, which is the opposite of myopia, or by presbyopia. Both hyperopia and presbyopia interfere with a person's ability to see things close-up. A farsighted person might have to hold a page at arm's length in order to read it.

What Makes the Eye See, and What Makes It See Incorrectly?

A person's ability to see depends on how well his or her eyes are able to bend light. When light enters the

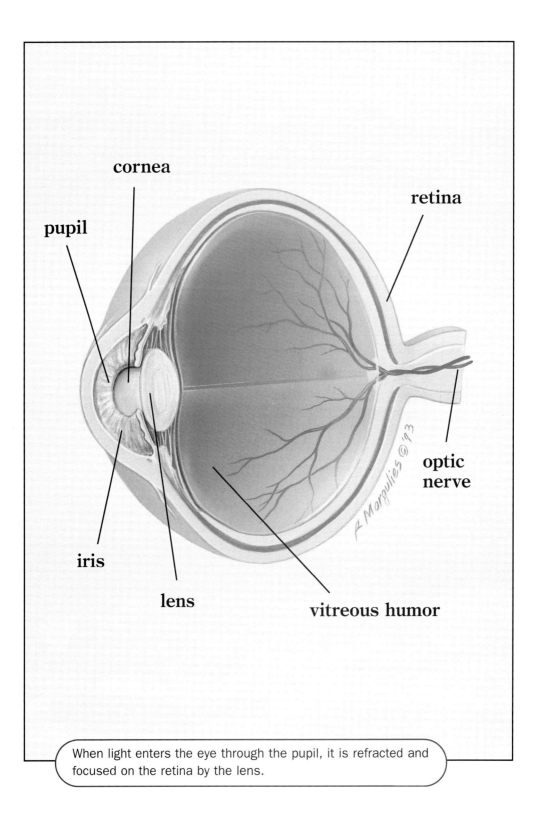

cornea

retina

pupil

iris

lens

vitreous humor

optic nerve

A Margulies ©'93

When light enters the eye through the pupil, it is refracted and focused on the retina by the lens.

eye, it is bent or "refracted" so that it becomes focused on the retina, which is the back, inside surface of the eye. Nearsightedness and farsightedness are both considered "refractive errors" because the light entering the eye is not being bent and focused exactly as it should.

You might think that the eyeball is a perfectly round sphere, but it is not. Nearsighted people's eyes are actually too long, so light from distant objects is focused in front of the retina. The eyes of people with hyperopia are too short, causing light from close objects to focus behind the retina.

Another common problem is called astigmatism. Astigmatism is blurred vision that is caused by having a cornea—the front layer of the eye that covers the lens and the colored iris—with an uneven surface. Some

What Does 20/20 Mean?

Vision that measures "20/20" is considered normal. If you have it, then you can see an object twenty feet away as well as other people with normal vision. This doesn't necessarily mean you can see the object clearly—just that you can see it as clearly as others with 20/20 vision. Vision that measures 20/40 means you can see at twenty feet what a person with normal vision can see at forty feet.

people with astigmatism might have a cornea that is wavy, which causes the light coming through it to go back to the retina in an uneven pattern.

Corrective Measures

Most cases of nearsightedness, farsightedness, and astigmatism can be corrected or at least improved with glasses or contact lenses. The choice between glasses or contacts is often a trade-off between vanity and expense. Many people, especially teens, don't want to wear glasses because they don't like the way glasses look. But glasses are generally less expensive than contacts. However, contacts make more sense for people who are very active or who need excellent peripheral, or side, vision.

As an alternative to glasses and contact lenses, surgery is sometimes performed to correct nearsightedness. The first form of surgery developed to correct myopia was radial keratotomy. This surgery involves cutting the cornea in a certain pattern to change its shape. Most often, though, surgery is not a good idea for teenagers because their eyes will continue to change, sometimes a lot, as they grow into adults. Getting new glasses twice a year may be expensive, but having surgery every six months is just not practical or safe.

If you believe you would like to have surgery to correct nearsightedness, do some research to learn everything you can about the different procedures. Then keep up with new developments in the field so that you will be well informed about your options when you are developed enough to enjoy the long-term benefits of the surgery.

Color Vision

Your ability to see colors comes from cells within the retina called cone cells. Cone cells and their partners, rod cells, work together to convert light that enters the eye into electrical impulses that travel back into the brain. These impulses appear to us as our visual images.

There are three different types of cone cells. Each type "sees" either red, green, or blue. Some people have defective cone cells. This condition, known as color-blindness, occurs in about 8 percent of males and less than 1 percent of females. Color-blindness, or more accurately, color vision deficiency, is almost never a large handicap. People who have it usually have trouble with reds and greens. It is extremely rare for a person to be unable to see any colors. While most cases of color vision deficiency are hereditary—it is passed from parents to children—some people develop it as they age because they are taking medication or because of an eye disease they contract.

Color vision deficiency is tested for in eye exams. The test might involve reading words created in a red-and-green design. A color-vision-deficient person will see different words than a person with correct color vision.

Sometimes people can have just a slight problem with one color, a problem so slight that it won't even register on the color-vision test. They might never even know they have it.

Opt...Opth...What?

The person who helps you with your vision will have one of three titles: optician, optometrist, or ophthalmologist (pronounced OP-tha-MOL-uh-jist). An ophthalmologist is a true "eye doctor" who can test your eyes, prescribe glasses or contacts, diagnose and treat eye diseases, and even perform surgery on your eyes. An optometrist is not a medical doctor, but he or she has graduated from a school of optometry and can test your vision and prescribe glasses or contacts. An optometrist can also detect signs of disease in the eye and can alert you to see an ophthalmologist. An optician is the person who fills the prescriptions for corrective lenses—glasses or contacts—written by optometrists and ophthalmologists. An optician creates the lenses for your glasses and fits them into the frames. If you get contact lenses, an optician makes sure that the lenses fit the unique shape of your eyeball. An optician does not examine your eyes or test your vision.

Chapter Two

Take Action: Don't Ignore These Problems

There are a lot of different health problems that can cause poor vision, but they don't have to. If you catch these problems before they go too far, you have a good chance of saving or improving your sight. There are some conditions that cause frightening symptoms in the eyes, but they do not permanently damage the eye. These conditions are also discussed here because they are your body's way of using your eyes to draw your attention to a problem somewhere else in your body.

Crossed Eyes and Lazy Eyes

When Lara's little brother, Andrew, was born, she was ecstatic. She had always wanted a baby brother or sister, and now she finally had one. Lara decorated the whole house in blue ribbons and balloons to welcome her mom and new baby brother home.

As soon as Lara held Andrew, she imagined teaching him to walk, talk, and read. Lara and her parents often found themselves standing over Andrew's crib for hours, just watching him wiggle and giggle. The whole family laughed at the way his eyes would move around in different directions, kind of like a lizard. Although Lara was worried, her mom told her that Andrew would outgrow it in a few months.

Unfortunately, six months later Andrew's eyes were still moving around without a lot of control. It was decided that Andrew should go to the doctor and get his eyes checked.

Although it is normal for a newborn baby to have eyes that are not fully developed, it was a good idea for Andrew to go to the doctor. At six months of age, he was getting too old to be experiencing the symptoms of a newborn. Luckily, the doctor informed Lara and her family that Andrew's eyesight was going to be fine.

Normally, a person's eyes move together and point in the same direction. If a person's eyes "cross," it seems like they are looking at their own nose. If instead of both turning inward, one eye turns outward, that is described as a "wall eye." Both of these conditions are known by the general term "strabismus."

A person with strabismus has eyes that are not working together to focus on what they see and then send a single picture back to the brain. Instead, each eye is sending its own version of what the person is looking at. This may cause the person to have blurred or double vision. This condition is very confusing for the brain. After a while, the brain will start to ignore the impulses that one eye is sending. The eye that is ignored will eventually become "lazy," or unused. The scientific term for "lazy eye" is "amblyopia" and if left untreated, the eye will actually become blind. In fact, amblyopia is the leading cause of single-eye blindness today.

Strabismus can be very hard to detect. Sometimes the flaw is so slight that you can't really even tell by just looking at the person. Still, even a slight misalignment can cause permanent problems. For this reason, it is very important to correct strabismus and amblyopia as soon as they are detected. Early detection can save the sight of the weaker eye. People who are blind in one eye can still see, but they lose an important ability called "depth perception," as well as a lot of peripheral vision.

Depth perception is what allows you to be able to tell how close an object is to you. Without depth perception, you might reach for something and expect to touch it, when in fact it is several inches away from your hand. You might have trouble going up and

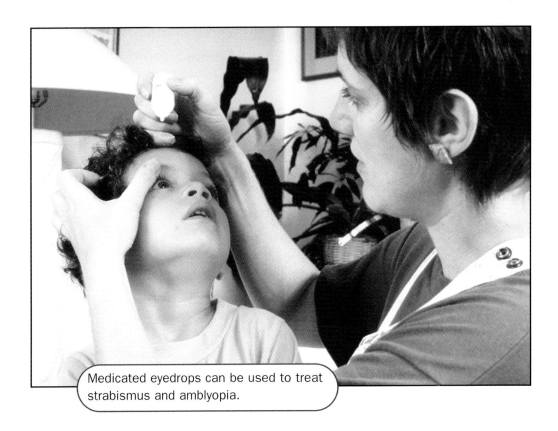

Medicated eyedrops can be used to treat strabismus and amblyopia.

down stairs because you can't tell how high or low to step. People with no depth perception have a very hard time playing sports that involve throwing and catching a ball.

Treatment for strabismus and amblyopia can include special glasses, an eyepatch, medicated eyedrops, eye exercises, or surgery. It is important that treatment begin as soon as possible, even before school-age, so that these conditions can be corrected immediately.

Signs of Trouble

Children can have other serious vision problems, and even their parents might not know. Here are some warning signs:

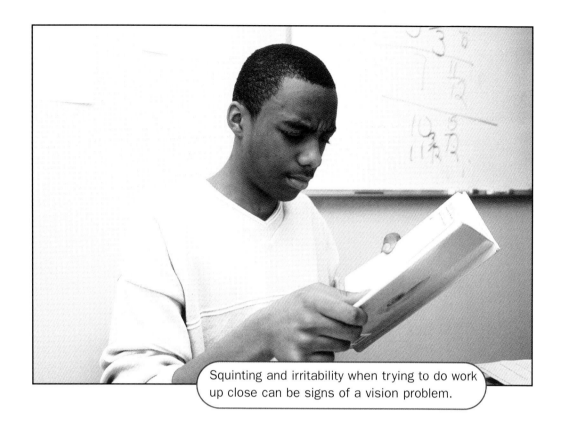

Squinting and irritability when trying to do work up close can be signs of a vision problem.

- Rubbing eyes excessively

- Covering or closing one eye

- Squinting or excessive blinking

- Frowning or irritability when trying to do work up close

- Holding objects very close to the eyes

Diabetic Retinopathy

Diabetic retinopathy occurs when small blood vessels in the retina begin to leak blood. Although new blood vessels do begin to grow in the retina, they are much weaker than they need to be. These weak vessels begin to trickle blood into the eyeball, which causes blurred vision.

Diabetic retinopathy often occurs in people who have diabetes. It is the leading cause of blindness in people under age sixty. In fact, diabetics are twenty-five times more likely to lose their sight than are nondiabetics. If caught in the early stages, diabetic retinopathy can be treated with laser surgery, which is why all diabetics should have frequent eye exams.

Glaucoma

Glaucoma is caused when there is too much pressure on the inside of the eyeball. A normal eye is filled with fluid that the body replaces on a regular basis. Glaucoma is caused when new fluid comes in faster than the old fluid can drain out, often because the drainage path is blocked. As pressure builds in the eye, blood flow to the retina and the optic nerve is cut off. The result of this is damaged vision or blindness.

Prevent Blindness America estimates that one in thirty people over age forty have glaucoma, and half of those people don't know they have it. In raw numbers, over two million Americans are affected by the disease. Fortunately, glaucoma can be treated if it is caught early. Treatment might include laser surgery or medication that lowers pressure within the eye and keeps the fluids at a safe level. Any sight that has been lost will not return, but treatment can prevent additional damage.

Sadly, about 120,000 people are blind as a result of glaucoma. The risk of blindness is another reason why it is so important for everyone to have regular eye exams. When you have an eye exam, you should be given a glaucoma test in which a machine sends a puff of air toward your eye. This test can be unnerving because the puff of air might startle you. However, not only is the test not painful, the air never actually touches your eye. Just knowing how important this test is should make it easy to tolerate.

Cataracts

For the past sixteen years, Heidi and her grand-mother have spent every other Sunday doing their artwork together. One Sunday afternoon, as the summer sun bounced off the windows, Heidi and her grandmother worked on their paintings.

As Heidi reached over to grab a different brush so she could define the outline of her clouded sky, she sneaked a look at her grandma's painting. "Grandma, are you doing an abstract piece?"

"Heidi, you know I do only realistic paintings. Why would you ask that?"

"Well, it's just that your fruit basket has blue apples and pink bananas. Not only that, but the painting looks smudged."

Cataract eye

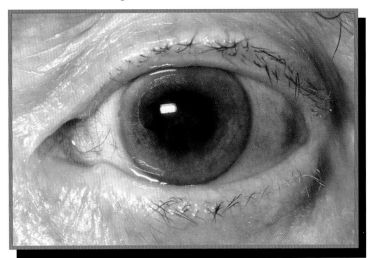

Normal eye

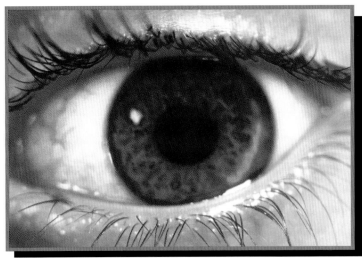

A cataract is a clouding of the lens of the eye. Usually, a cataract is developed with age.

"Really? I knew that lately everything looked foggy, but I was hoping it would just pass. I'll call for an eye appointment on Monday."

Two weeks later, Heidi sat in the sky blue waiting room of the hospital and hoped her grandmother would get out of surgery soon. The doctors had promised that cataract surgery is a common procedure and that her grandmother would regain all of her sight.

Heidi's grandmother was experiencing cataracts. A cataract is a cloudy area in the lens of the eye. It can happen in one or both eyes, and in most instances a cataract develops with age. As a person gets older, the lenses of the eyes simply start to wear out. The National Alliance for Eye and Vision Research estimates that about 29 percent of all people between the ages of sixty-five and seventy-four have cataracts. Young people can also get cataracts, though then it is the result of an injury, eye infection, or a disease.

Just like Heidi's grandmother described it, looking through a cataract is like seeing the world through a gray fog or mist. Over time, though, cataracts tend to grow worse. When the cataract starts to interfere with a person's vision enough to reduce his or her quality of life, surgery is usually recommended. The surgeon removes the cloudy lens and replaces it with something similar to a permanent contact lens.

The information Heidi received from the doctor was accurate—cataract surgery has become very common and is almost always successful. Cataracts used to cause thousands of cases of blindness every year, but now that surgery is more reliable and less feared, cataracts do not have to lead to permanent loss of sight.

Retinitis Pigmentosa

This condition is hereditary, and it causes the retina to break down. It can begin in childhood. The first sign of retinitis pigmentosa is poor night vision, followed by the loss of peripheral vision. Eventually, this condition results in tunnel vision, a condition in which a person can see only straight ahead through a small area of the eye. A person who has retinitis pigmentosa to the extent that he or she has tunnel vision is considered legally blind.

Retinitis pigmentosa affects approximately 100,000 Americans and is the leading cause of blindness from an inherited condition. Currently, there is no treatment. However, the National Alliance for Eye and Vision Research reports that progress has been made to identify the causes of this disease, which could eventually lead to the development of a treatment.

High Blood Pressure

High blood pressure, or hypertension, can cause bleeding in the retina. This can lead to a scarred retina,

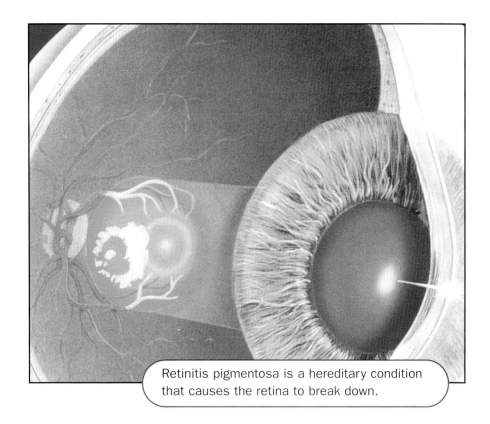

Retinitis pigmentosa is a hereditary condition that causes the retina to break down.

which will damage your vision. People with high blood pressure might have changes in the retina and still have normal vision. However, these changes are still important because they alert the ophthalmologist to possible problems in other parts of the body. The kidneys and heart are especially susceptible to damage from high blood pressure, and problems with your eyes can help lead to the discovery of other problems.

Papilledema

Papilledema is the death of the optic nerve. It is usually caused by increased pressure inside the skull, which can result from high blood pressure or from a growth in the brain. As the optic nerve is squeezed, vision slowly becomes poor. Vision can be restored if this condition is treated in time.

Macular Degeneration

There is an area in the retina that contains a great number of rod and cone cells. This area is called the macula, and it allows you to see fine details such as small print or a tiny splinter in your finger. As people age, the macula sometimes breaks down, which causes them to lose sight in the center of their field of vision.

Approximately 1.7 million people suffer from decreased vision as a result of macular degeneration, and 100,000 are blind from the disease. Some people with the disease find that they are still able to read through the use of powerful magnifiers. Macular degeneration is painless and generally develops slowly. In some cases, it is partially treatable, and promising research may make it possible to transplant healthy cells to restore sight. Again, regular eye exams allow for early treatment and give the best chance of saving the person's sight.

Cancer

Cancer that affects the eyes or the brain can damage or destroy vision. One form of cancer that affects the eyes is called retinoblastoma. Again, if it is treated in time, vision can be saved.

Melanoma, a cancer that usually grows on the skin and is believed to be related to overexposure to the sun, can also occur in the eyes. This form of cancer may also be treatable, depending on where in the eye it occurs and how advanced it is when it is discovered. These are just two of the many forms of cancer that can affect vision. As with most diseases, early detection is the key to reducing potential damage.

Other Eye Symptoms

These conditions usually do not damage a person's vision. However, each one could be a sign of a serious health problem, and some could lead to vision problems if left untreated. If you have one of these conditions, talk to an adult—a parent, your doctor, the school nurse—and make sure it's nothing serious.

- Black eye. Besides the bruise you see, there could be more damage inside, such as internal bleeding or a fractured bone.

- Dark circles under eye. This could be from lack of sleep, stress, or just from having delicate skin in the eye area. It may also be something more serious, such as allergies or anemia (too little iron in the blood), so if the dark circles last a long time, see a doctor.

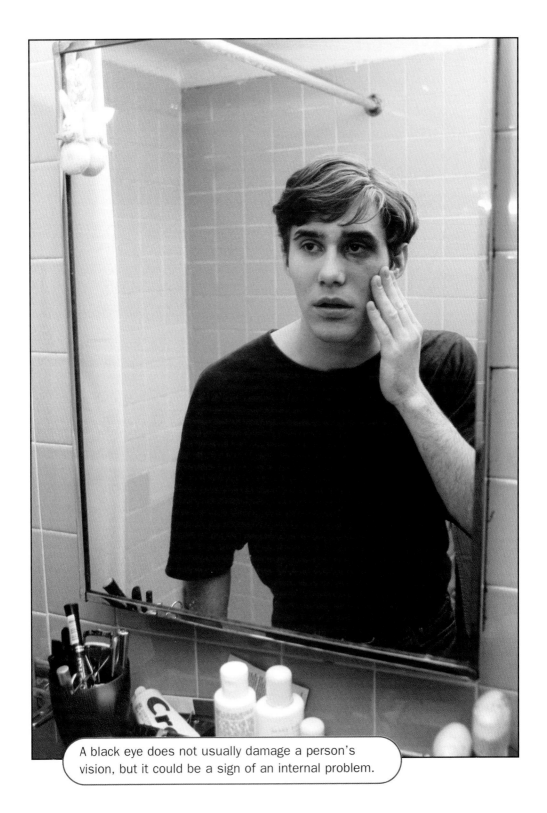

A black eye does not usually damage a person's vision, but it could be a sign of an internal problem.

- Itchy or painful eye. This could indicate an eye infection, especially if the eye is watering excessively or if there is pus. If your eyes are itchy and watery, and you arc sneezing and have a runny nose, you might have allergies.

- Headache and pain in eyes. If you have a very severe headache that causes your eyes to hurt and makes you sensitive to light, you might have a migraine or cluster headache. Cluster headaches are short but painful headaches that usually cause intense pain in the eyes. Migraines, on the other hand, last for a longer amount of time, but most often their pain is less intense.

- Blood spot in eye. If you find a small spot of blood in the white part of your eye, it means one of the tiny blood vessels of the eye has ruptured. This can be caused by a blow to the eye or even by coughing, vomiting, or sneezing. It can also indicate something more serious. If you get one of these spots and you can think of no reason for it, you should see a doctor.

- Yellow eyes. If the whites of your eyes are turning yellow, get to your doctor right away. This is almost always a sign of a serious liver problem.

What Is "Blindness"?

You might think that "blindness" means that a person can't see anything. That is one form of blindness, but there are others.

When vision breaks down past a certain point, the person is considered "legally blind." He or she might see well enough to care for himself or herself, but not well enough to drive, read a book, work on a computer, or use household tools. According to the National Association for Visually Handicapped, approximately 1.3 million Americans are considered legally blind, and approximately 10 percent of those people are completely sightless or can see only a slight amount of light.

People who are legally blind—but not completely blind—are still able to see light and dark, but they cannot make out details. This condition is also called "low vision." There are many tools and devices available to help people with low vision, including many different types of magnifiers that enable them to read a book or to see the images on a television or computer screen. There are also organizations to help people with low vision, such as the National Association for Visually Handicapped.

A person might also be blind in just one eye. This is called monocular blindness. As we discussed earlier, since the eyes normally work together to give you depth perception, people who become blind in one eye will have trouble knowing how near or far they are from objects that they see.

A person can also be color-blind, or color vision deficient. Remember, people who are color vision deficient usually have trouble telling the difference between reds and greens, although a rarer form affects how a person sees blues and yellows. The condition affects males much more often than females.

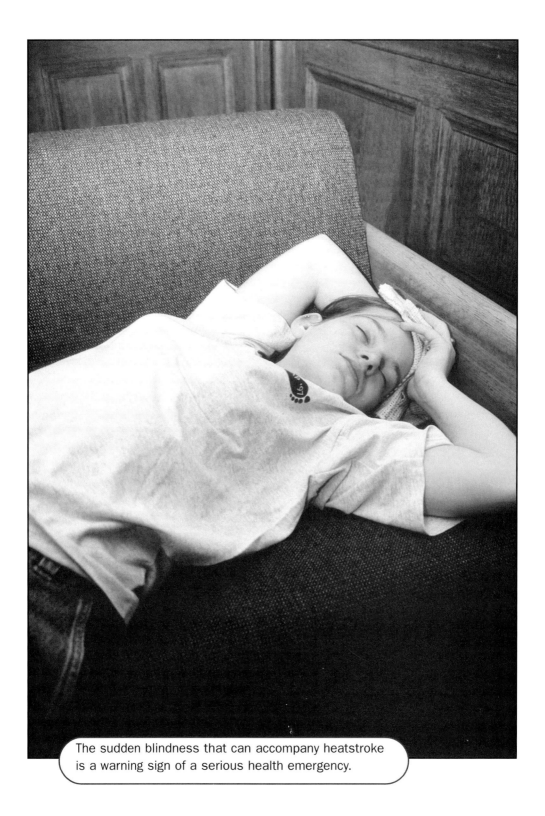

The sudden blindness that can accompany heatstroke is a warning sign of a serious health emergency.

Chapter Three

Emergency! Get Help Now

The conditions described in this chapter are all emergencies. If you or someone you know experiences these symptoms, go to a hospital immediately.

Sudden Blindness

Maria was at softball practice one summer morning, playing first base. It was really hot and she had skipped breakfast. She wasn't feeling too great, and even though she was really thirsty, she decided not to disrupt practice to get a drink.

All of a sudden, Maria couldn't see. It was like there was an orange-brown film over her eyes. Somebody threw the ball to her and it hit her: She had no idea it was coming. The coach ran over. When she moved really close to Maria's face, Maria could see her, but just barely. The coach made Maria drink a lot of cold water and then had her sit in the shade of a tree. Maria's mother was called so Maria could be taken to the emergency room.

After being treated, Maria could see again, but she was completely out of it. It wasn't until the next morning, after having a good dinner and a long, sound sleep, that Maria felt normal again.

Maria was suffering from heatstroke, a potentially life-threatening condition that is common on very hot, humid days. In this case, the combination of hot weather, exercise, skipping breakfast, and going without water led up to this dangerous situation. In a way, the temporary blindness that came with the heatstroke was a good thing: It made it impossible for Maria to ignore the fact that her body needed rest, food, and fluids. She knew that she didn't feel well, but she tried to "play through it." When she suddenly couldn't see, she and the coach knew to take the situation seriously.

If you ever experience blurred or double vision, your vision clouds over, or you find you can't see, even in just part of your field of vision, go to the emergency room. Don't wait for the symptoms to go away on their own. They might not go away. Maria may not have known any better, but she should have taken better care of herself and told the coach about her symptoms immediately.

Detached Retina

Sudden blindness can also be a sign of a detached retina. The retina can actually peel away from its place in the back of the inside of the eye, causing the person to see a shower of sparks or what seems like a curtain being pulled across part or all of his or her field of vision. Retinal detachment is often the result of a head injury, but it can happen without any obvious cause. If it is caught in time and the victim receives immediate surgery, the retina can usually be reattached successfully. If the retina is not reattached, or if too much time passes and the cells in the retina have time to die, the person will have permanent loss of sight. Never ignore signs such as flashing lights or blank areas in your field of vision.

Impact Injuries

According to Prevent Blindness America, car accidents are the leading cause of eye injuries in young children. However, no matter what the situation, anything that hits you in the head or face has the potential to harm your vision.

See a doctor any time your head has suffered a hard hit, especially if you black out or feel dizzy or confused afterward. If there is any bleeding, or if you have any visual disturbances such as double vision, blurred vision, flashing lights, floating spots, or blank or dark areas in your field of vision, you might have a concussion or a

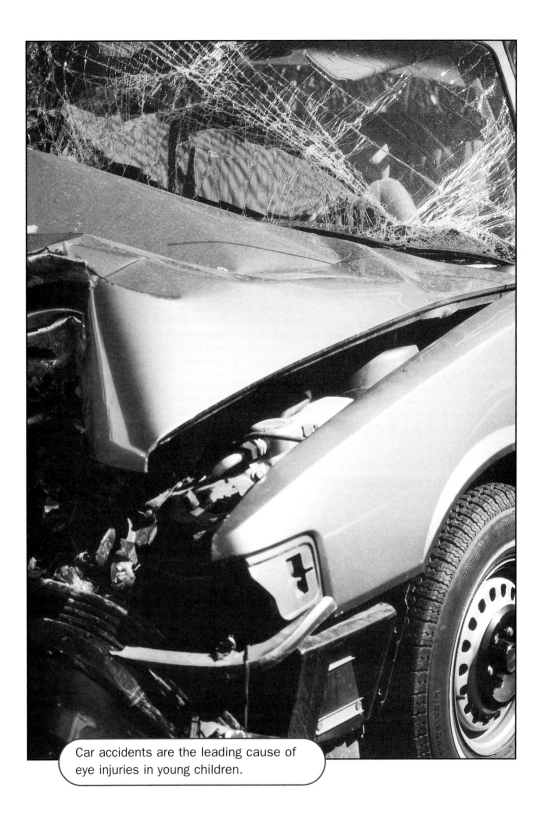

Car accidents are the leading cause of eye injuries in young children.

skull fracture. Both of these injuries must be treated and monitored for complications. The same is true of any injury to your eyes: If something pokes you in the eye, you should see a doctor to check for scratches on your cornea. If an object is embedded in your eye, do not pull it out. You should carefully cover both of your eyes (even if only one is hurt) to prevent them from moving, and then have someone take you to an emergency room immediately.

Burns

You might have heard that you can damage your eyes by looking directly into the sun, even during an eclipse. This is true. Never look directly at the sun or an eclipse, even for a second. You might think you can peek at it, and when you find that it doesn't hurt right away, you might be tempted to look longer. Unfortunately, even if it doesn't hurt right away, you might still be damaging your retinas, and it will eventually hurt them very badly. Looking at the sun through a telescope will cause even more severe damage.

Chemical burns are also dangerous to your sight. If you ever accidentally splash a chemical in your eyes, get help immediately to prevent permanent damage.

Don't Open That Eye

If someone's eye has been injured and it is swollen shut, do not attempt to force it open to get a better look.

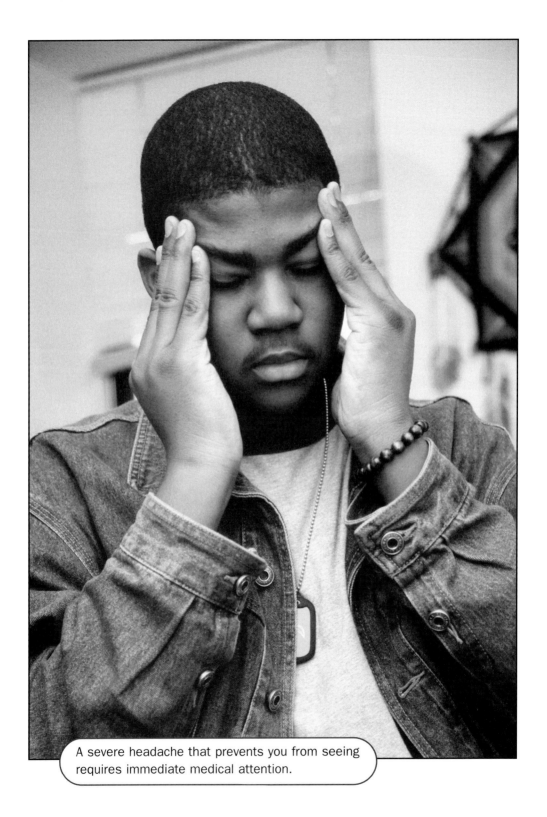

A severe headache that prevents you from seeing requires immediate medical attention.

There may be injuries or cuts to the eyeball that will be made worse if the eye is opened. Get to an emergency room as fast as possible.

Vision Emergencies

Go to the emergency room immediately if you have any of these symptoms:

- You see flashes of light and floating black shapes, or halos around lights.

- It seems like a curtain is being drawn across your field of vision.

- You have a severe headache that makes it difficult or impossible for you to see.

- Light hurts your eyes so badly that you can't stand to open them.

- You suddenly have blurred or double vision, or some areas of your field of vision seem blocked or distorted.

- Your eyes begin to bulge out or cross.

- You have severe pain in one or both eyes.

- You have something stuck in your eye.

- You suddenly can't see or have very diminished sight.

Chapter Four

Protecting Your Sight

Many cases of blindness and impaired vision are not preventable. If you are nearsighted, for example, there's nothing you could have done to prevent it. However, most injuries and infections can be avoided and many of the diseases that cause poor vision or blindness can be controlled or avoided. Here are some tips on protecting your sight.

Preventing Infections

When the alarm clock sounded its loud music, Jana hit the snooze button and rolled back over to savor a few more minutes of sleep. Five minutes later, she heard the banging music again.

"Ugh, Mondays are so gross," she complained. But when she tried to open her eyes, only one

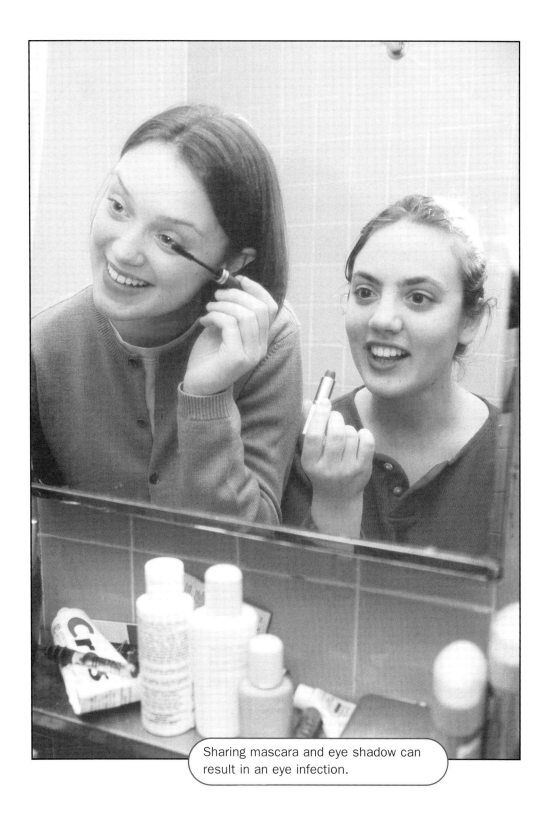

Sharing mascara and eye shadow can result in an eye infection.

would open. She lifted her hand and felt that her right eye was covered with gunk.

When Jana walked into the kitchen a few minutes later, her mother stood at the counter drinking her morning cup of coffee.

"Mom, I have another eye infection. Call the doctor, will you?"

"Jana, you have to stop sharing makeup with your friends. You have had six eye infections this year, and all of them are because you insist on sharing mascara and eye shadow."

"I know. It's just that Erin works at the Clinique counter at the mall, so she always has the best makeup. I have to try all the colors, Mom."

"Well, why don't we go to the mall today and you can pick out a few colors that you like. But that means you can use only your own makeup from now on."

Jana was suffering from pink eye, also called conjunctivitis, which is a very contagious eye infection. Although treatable, pink eye can be painful. As Jana's mother stressed to her, sharing makeup is one of the easiest ways to contract pink eye and other eye infections. For this reason, you should also never share handkerchiefs, eye drops, contact lenses, or contact lens cases or solutions. All of these items, and any others

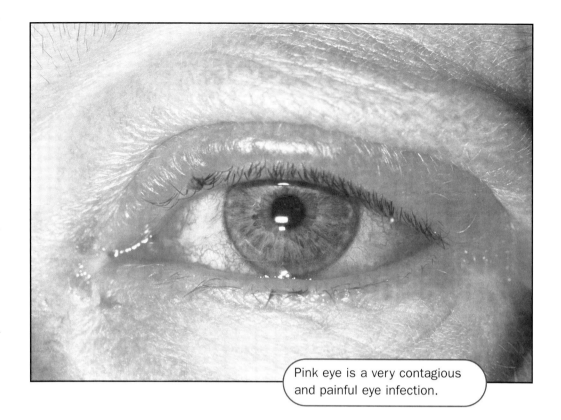

Pink eye is a very contagious and painful eye infection.

that people commonly touch their eyes with, can spread germs, even if the other person does not appear to have an infection.

Eye infections can harm your sight if they become very severe. The most important thing you can do to prevent eye infections is to avoid touching or rubbing your eyes. When you touch your eyes, you risk transferring germs from your fingers into your eyes and giving yourself an eye infection or a cold. If you must touch your eyes, for example, if you wear contacts, be sure to wash your hands first.

If you wear contact lenses, be sure to clean them regularly. Experts suggest that you never wear your contacts to sleep. If you have disposable contacts, throw them away after the number of days recommended by the manufacturer and be sure to keep them clean.

Avoiding Injuries

Prevent Blindness America estimates that 90 percent of all eye injuries could be prevented or made less severe if people knew more about common eye dangers. One example is sports-related injuries, which account for 40,000 trips to the emergency room each year. Anyone who plays baseball, basketball, and racquet sports is especially vulnerable to eye injuries.

How to Choose Protective Eyewear

Prevent Blindness America reports that almost all eye injuries could have been prevented by wearing the right eye protection. Here are some tips on choosing protective eyewear:

- Sports require the strongest eye protection. Regular glasses and even workshop safety glasses are not enough to protect the eyes from a lot of sports injuries.

- Workshop safety glasses are available from home-improvement stores. Be sure to choose a pair that provides full protection for your eyes and that are specifically intended to protect you when you use tools.

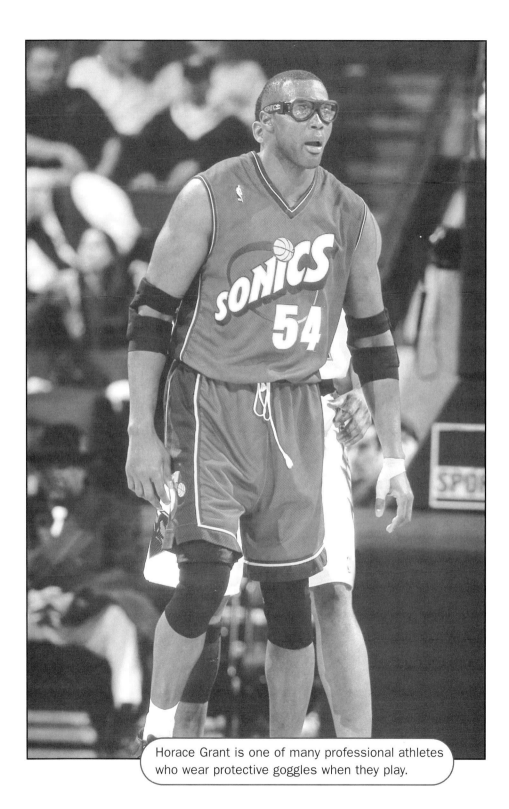
Horace Grant is one of many professional athletes who wear protective goggles when they play.

- Make sure that the eyeguards you choose have the lenses already in them and that the lenses are designed to either stay in place or pop outward.

- If you are concerned about foggy lenses, check out eyeguards that have an antifog coating or that have vents on the sides to allow air to circulate.

- Be sure to choose an eyeguard that is made of polycarbonate material because it is the most impact-resistant material available.

- Make sure that the eye protector you choose has padding on the areas that touch your face, including the top ridge and the nose piece. This padding will keep the eyeguard from cutting you if you are hit hard.

- Make sure your eyeguard fits properly. Ask for help from someone at a store who is familiar with the various products and can help you find the right size.

Home Injuries

A common location where eye injuries occur is the home. In fact, since safety regulations must now be followed in the workplace, the home has become the fastest growing location for eye injuries. Toys and home playground equipment cause over 11,000 eye injuries every year.

Toys with sharp pointed ends, like darts, and toys that shoot things can do the most serious damage. Paintball guns, slingshots, and other toys that propel objects at high speeds are also very dangerous and should be used with great care. BB guns, bow-and-arrow sets, and hunting guns are weapons and should be used only in a range or area that is blocked off specifically for their use. Even then, only after sufficient training and with supervision should you use such items. Fireworks are also dangerous no matter how careful you are. If you are determined to play with fireworks, do it only with adult supervision and be sure to wear eye protection.

Injuries in the home can also happen when children or their parents are cleaning or working on projects. The chemicals that are used to clean a house, wash clothes or dishes, fertilize plants, kill bugs, treat swimming pool water, or strip paint can all be very dangerous to the eyes. Always wear eye protection when working with or around these chemicals. You should always wear eye protection when working in a science lab or playing with a home science kit. Before working with a chemical, such as a household cleaner, read the label for instructions about what to do if you get the chemical in your eyes.

The use of tools in a home workshop or for yard work can also put the eyes at risk. Whenever you work

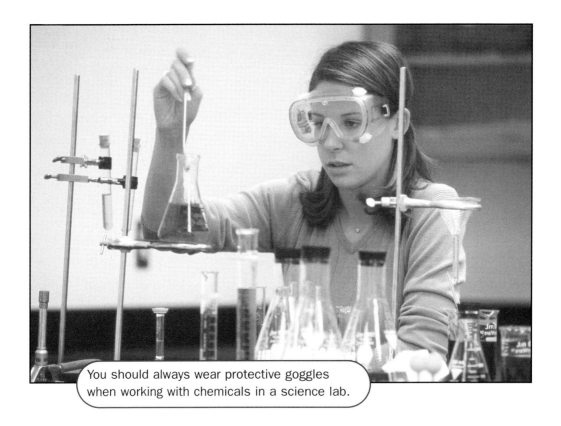

You should always wear protective goggles when working with chemicals in a science lab.

with tools, whether they are hand tools, power tools, or even yard machines such as lawnmowers, you should have adult supervision. Never use tools that are too big or that are beyond your ability to control. If you have to reach up to grasp the handle of a lawnmower, or if you cannot handle a tool properly, you should not use it. Allow someone else to handle these tasks for the time being.

Dealing with Diseases

As you have already read, there are a large number of diseases that can lead to poor vision or blindness. But the damage from these conditions can be prevented or reduced with early detection and proper medical care.

The single most important thing you can do to protect your sight is to have regular eye exams. Many people think they need to go to the eye doctor only if they need glasses or contacts, or if they have corrective lenses and need their prescription updated. This is not true, as you now know. Again, be sure to tell your parents, grandparents, and other family members about what you have read in this book, and encourage them to have regular eye exams. Many of the eye problems discussed here are more common among older people. By warning them of the dangers, you can help them to keep their vision.

Remember, if you have any sudden changes in your vision or if you experience any troubling symptoms such as pain, double vision, blurred vision, flashes of light, recurring headaches, or blank spots in your field of vision, get to a doctor right away.

Vision Myths

Myth: Don't read in poor light. You'll strain your eyes.

Fact: The phrase "eye strain" implies that you can hurt your eyes by using them too much. This is not true. You can give yourself a headache and make your eyes tired with too much reading, too much time on the computer, or too much time playing video games, especially if the lights in the room are not bright enough. However, these activities won't actually harm your vision.

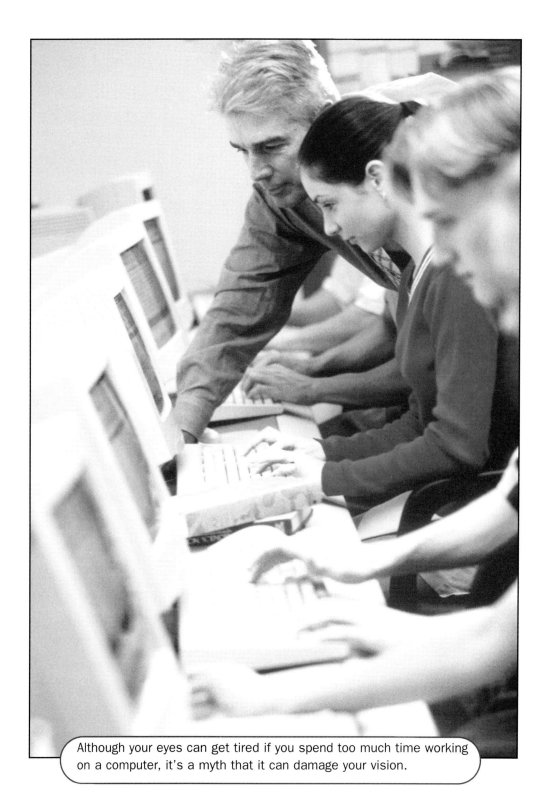

Although your eyes can get tired if you spend too much time working on a computer, it's a myth that it can damage your vision.

Myth: If you can't see very well, don't try to use your eyes. Save your sight.

Fact: It is not true that people who have poor vision should try not to use their eyes too much. In fact, the opposite is true. The National Association for Visually Handicapped says that people with impaired vision should continue to use their eyesight as much as possible or the brain might "forget" how to see and cause them to lose even more of their sight.

Myth: Eating carrots will give you better vision.

Fact: It is true that carrots contain vitamin A, which is important for good vision, but you don't need to eat tons of carrots to get enough vitamin A. In fact, taking in too much vitamin A (usually caused by taking supplements) can damage your body. Also, carrots are not the only source of vitamin A; it is also found in leafy green vegetables and in cantaloupe.

Myth: If you cross your eyes, they might stay that way.

Fact: This is completely untrue. Crossing your eyes does strain them and could give you a headache. But crossing your eyes is not going to cause them to remain that way.

You now know what you can do to protect your sight, both from injuries and from disease. While there are some conditions that you can't control or avoid, such as nearsightedness or farsightedness, there are many others that you can prevent or make less severe by taking good care of your eyes and your overall health. You now know that one of the best ways to prevent eye problems is to have regular eye exams. You also know how to help others to protect themselves, by reminding them to wear eye protection and by being careful not to endanger another person's sight through dangerous play or the careless use of tools.

If you would like to learn even more about the topics discussed here, check out the books and Web sites in the For Further Reading and Where to Go for Help sections at the end of this book.

Most people take their vision for granted until it is damaged or lost. But with a little bit of attention to prevention and care, you can increase your chances of having good vision throughout your life.

Glossary

amblyopia   A condition that can result from strabismus, in which one eye is weaker than the other and needs to be forced to work correctly; also called a "lazy eye."

astigmatism   A problem caused by an uneven cornea surface that can affect how well you see.

cataract   A clouding of the lens of an eye.

color-blindness   The common term for color vision deficiency, in which a person is unable to correctly see colors.

cone cells   The cells in the retina that are responsible for "reading" light and color.

conjunctivitis   A common eye infection also known as pink eye.

cornea   The front layer of the eye that lies over the lens and the iris.

depth perception The ability to judge distances between yourself and objects you see. You must have the
use of both eyes to have accurate depth perception.

diabetes A disease that can cause serious complications in the eyes that can lead to blindness.

diabetic retinopathy A complication of diabetes
that can damage the retinas and cause blindness.

farsightedness A vision problem that prevents the
person from seeing things clearly close-up.

glaucoma A disease caused by increased pressure
within the eye that can lead to poor vision
or blindness.

hypertension The formal name for high blood pressure, which can cause eye problems.

iris The colored ring of tissue behind the cornea and in
front of the lens; regulates the amount of light entering the eye by adjusting the size of the pupil.

lens The middle part of the eye through which
light enters.

macula The portion of the retina that allows you to
see fine detail.

macular degeneration A condition in which the
macula breaks down, causing the person to lose
sight in the center of his or her field of vision.

melanoma A form of cancer that sometimes occurs
in the eyes.

monocular Something that affects or involves only
one eye.

nearsightedness A vision problem that prevents the person from clearly seeing things from a distance; also called myopia.

optic nerve Bundle of over one million nerve fibers that carry visual messages from the retina to the brain.

papilledema Atrophy or death of the optic nerve, caused by excessive pressure inside the skull.

polycarbonate The strongest, most impact-resistant material available for eyeguards.

pupil The adjustable opening at the center of the iris that allows varying amounts of light to enter the eye.

radial keratotomy A surgical procedure used to correct nearsightedness.

retina The back, inside lining of the eye.

retinitis pigmentosa A hereditary condition that causes the retina to break down and can result in tunnel vision.

retinoblastoma A form of cancer of the eye.

rod cells Cells in the retina that "read" light coming into the eye.

strabismus A condition in which the eyes do not work together, causing crossed eyes, "wall eye," or other misalignments.

tunnel vision Being able to see only a small area, straight ahead, in the center of the field of vision.

vitreous humor The transparent mass of gel that lies behind the lens in front of the retina.

Where to Go for Help

In the United States

AMD Alliance International
11460 Johns Creek Parkway
Duluth, GA 30097
(877) 263-7171

American Council of the Blind
1155 15th Street NW
Suite 1004
Washington, DC 20005
(800) 424-8666
Web site: http://www.acb.org

National Alliance for Eye and Vision Research
426 C St. NE
Washington, DC 20002
(202) 544-1880
Web site: http://www.eyeresearch.org

National Association for Visually Handicapped
22 West 21st Street
New York, NY 10010
(212) 889-3141
E-mail: staff@navh.org
Web site: http://www.navh.org

National Cancer Institute
Office of Cancer Communications
31 Center Drive, MSC 2580
Bethesda, MD 20892-2580
(800) 422-6237
Web site: http://www.nci.nih.gov

Prevent Blindness America (formerly National
        Society to Prevent Blindness)
(800) 331-2020
E-mail: info@preventblindness.org
Web site: http://www.preventblindness.org

In Canada

The Canadian National Institute for the Blind
The CNIB Library for the Blind
1929 Bayview Avenue
Toronto, ON M4G 3E8
(800) 268-8818
Web site: http://www.cnib.ca

Foundation Fighting Blindness—Canada
Suite 910
36 Toronto Street
Toronto, ON M5C 2C5
(800) 461-3331
E-mail: info@rpresearch.ca
Web site: http//www.rpresearch.ca

The National Federation of the Blind
Suite 107
1455 Ellis Street
Kelowna, BC V1Y 2A3
(800) 561-4774
E-mail: nfbae@home.com
Web site: http://www.nfbae.ca

For Further Reading

Draughton, Henry. *Student's Vision Guide.* Garland, TX: Family Talk Incorporated, 1995.

Goldstein, Margaret J. *Eyeglasses.* Minneapolis, MN: Carolrhoda, 1996.

Landau, Elaine. *Blindness.* New York: Twenty-First Century Books Incorporated, 1995.

Olsen, Mary M., and Kenneth R. Harris. *Color Vision Deficiency and Color Blindness.* Eugene, OR: Fern Ridge Press, 1998.

Royal National Institute for the Blind. *Seeing a Future: Coming to Terms with Sight Loss.* London: Royal National Institute for the Blind, 1997.

Schaughnessy, Diane. *Let's Talk about Needing Glasses.* New York: Rosen Publishing Group, 1997.

Westcott, Patsy. *Living with Blindness.* Austin, TX: Raintree Steck-Vaughn, 1999.

Index

A
aging and vision, 15, 25, 28, 51
allergies, 29, 31
amblyopia, 19–20
anemia, 29
astigmatism, 13–14

B
blindness, 6, 7, 19, 22, 23, 26, 28,
    32–33, 42, 50
  legal, 26, 32
  monocular, 32–33
  sudden, 35–37, 41
blood pressure, high, 26–27
brain, 6, 15, 16, 19, 28, 53

C
cancer, 28–29
cataracts, 23–26
color-blindness (color vision
    deficiency), 15–16, 33
cone cells, 15, 28

contact lenses, 10, 14, 16, 25, 44,
    45–46, 51
cornea, 12, 13, 14, 39

D
diabetic retinopathy, 21–22

E
eye
  black, 29
  blood spot in, 31
  lazy, 19
  object embedded in, 39, 41
  wall, 18
eye disease, 6, 15, 16, 50, 53
  treatment for, 22–23, 26, 28, 29
eye exams (tests), 15, 16, 22, 23,
    28, 51, 54
eye infections, 25, 42, 44–45
eye injury, 6, 25, 37, 39, 42, 46, 53
  car accidents and, 37
  chemicals and, 49

Index

fireworks and, 49
head injury and, 37, 38–39
at home, 48–49
science labs and, 49
sports and, 20, 46
sun and, 39
tools and, 49–50, 54
toys and, 49
weapons and, 49
eye problems, treatment for, 7,
    20, 22–23, 26, 28, 29
eyes
    crossed, 17–18, 41, 53
    dark circles under, 29
    how they work, 11–13
    itchy, 31
    yellow, 31
eye surgery, 16, 20, 37
    cataract, 25–26
    laser, 22
    teens and, 14–15
eyewear, protective (eyeguards),
    46–48, 49, 54

F
farsightedness, 11, 13, 14, 53
flashing lights, 37, 41, 51

G
glasses, 10, 14, 16, 20, 46, 51
    teens and, 9–11, 14
glaucoma, 22–23

H
headaches, 31, 41, 51, 53
heatstroke, 36
hereditary problems, 15, 26
hyperopia, 11

I
iris, 12, 13

L
lens, 12, 13, 25
light, 11, 13, 14, 15, 32
    sensitivity to, 31, 41

M
macular degeneration, 28
magnifiers, 28, 32
melanoma, 29
myopia, 11, 14

N
National Association for Visually
    Handicapped, 32, 53
nearsightedness, 10, 11, 13, 14,
    42, 53

O
ophthalmologist, 16, 27
optician, 16
optic nerve, 12, 22, 27–28
optometrist, 16

P
papilledema, 27
pink eye (conjunctivitis), 44
presbyopia, 11
Prevent Blindness America, 22,
    37, 46
pupil, 12

R
radial keratotomy, 14
retina, 12, 13, 14, 15, 21, 22, 26,
    27, 28, 39
    detached, 37
retinitis pigmentosa, 26
retinoblastoma, 28
rod cells, 15, 28

S
strabismus, 18–20

T
20/20 vision, 13

V
vision
  blank areas in, 37, 51
  blurred, 19, 22, 36, 37, 41

depth perception, 19, 33
double, 19, 36, 41, 51
low, 32
myths about, 51–53
peripheral, 14, 19, 26
tunnel, 26
vision problems, signs of, 20–21
vitreous humor, 12

About the Author

Debbie Stanley has a bachelor's degree in journalism and a master's in industrial/organizational psychology.

Photo Credits

Cover by Ira Fox. Pp. 2, 8, 21, 30, 34, 40, 43 by Ira Fox; pp. 12, 20, 24, 27, 45 © Custom Medical; pp. 38, 52 © Superstock; p. 47 © Jed Jacobsohn/Allsport; p. 50 © Robert Llewellyn/Pictor.

Layout

Geri Giordano